My Pain Alert™ Scale

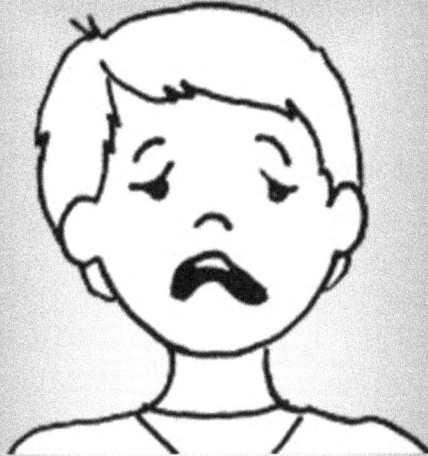

Communication Tool

By Gail Goldstein CCC - SLP
Jan Schippits and Blair Malloy

My Pain Alert ™ Scale Communication Tool

By Gail Goldstein, CCC-SLP - Speech Language Pathologist and Researcher

Jan Schippits - Marketing, Illustration and Design Consultant

Blair Malloy - Music, Consumer Use and Photography Consultant

Goldstein, Schippits and Malloy Media LLC

Copyright 2016 Gail Goldstein

Goldstein, Schippits and Malloy Media LLC

Richmond, KY 40475-7601 USA

www.mypainalert.com

ISBN print edition: 978-0-9981610-0-6

ISBN e-book edition: 978-0-9981610-1-3

Dedicated to Connor and all people who have dealt with pain for as long as they can remember.

Contents

How to Use

My Pain Alert ™ Scale

Communication Tool

My Pain Alert ™ Scale is a pain communication tool for parents and caregivers coping with loved ones in pain. Just as we train our children to communicate their bowel and bladder needs we can train them to communicate their pain. All children and adults with limited communication skills do and will experience pain. They need a tool to help them quickly and efficiently indicate their sensations. Your limited communicator needs to develop the skills to use a pain scale as a tool to get what they need. This requires practice. The tool they use needs to be easily understood, accessible and engaging. My Pain Alert ™ Scale should help them participate in their medical care.

My Pain Alert ™ Scale is appropriate for individuals with yes/no capability including: young children, autistic individuals, hearing impaired, vision impaired, neurologically impaired, and those with other forms of restricted communication. Anyone experiencing pain can use this tool.

Children's picture books or video either don't have characters in pain, or don't show a normal response to pain. Our ordinary environment has little to show the limited communicator how to deal with pain. The My Pain Alert ™ Scale pictures a boy with belly pain illustrating levels zero and one through five. When pain happens: first there is pain, then improvement as medication takes effect, then pain as the medication's effect fades with time in a down - up - down - up - down pattern. Zero indicates the person is fine and is located above levels two and three, as that is how pain is experienced. It makes sense to someone without formal mathematical training.

The training materials in sections two, three, and four are for caregivers to read to and with the limited communicator. Each level has text explaining it and helping relate it to their own experience. Repeated practice leads to better understanding and use of the scale. The caregiver can make each practice session about a different pain: headache, toothache, muscle pain, fever, pain from skin tears or bruises, and so on. Acting the part is encouraged. American Sign Language may be more accessible than speech for an individual, or may just be interesting learning. Use several practice sessions to try signing responses. The song, "Are You Hurting?" is intended to reach the visually impaired or musically driven. The distinct vowel sounds paired with each level are responses achievable by many verbally apraxic individuals. The refrain is designed to alert the individual that now is their special time to communicate how they are feeling.

Fifteen minutes is a good length of time for one practice session. Once there is some reliability, it is still good to review My Pain Alert ^{TM} materials periodically with a person who is a limited communicator. Refer to Brief Annotated Bibliography for ideas as to how much practice may be needed.

Using all the senses helps the learning process. Limited communicators and the very young may have strengths in: seeing, listening, pointing, signing, visual tracking, gesturing, mimicking, vocalizing, repeating, telling, or singing. Varying the method of responding to the materials makes the repeat telling of each level interesting. Stressing one input or output method during each practice session can help clarify what methods work best for the individual. Caregivers should determine the individual's best ways to take information in and get responses out. Practice data recorded by caregivers may help medical professionals be efficient and accurate in their care. See "Caregiver Notes to Support Medical Care" for a recording method which is simple and quick. Since the individual already struggles to get their thoughts across, make the use of the My Pain Alert ^{TM} Scale as easy for them as possible.

Discussion and personalization are encouraged. Use the limited communicator's people network. Who might give a pinch or a hug? Who would give medicine? Relate the stories to their life. Does Grandpa hurt? What picture would Grandpa use to show his pain? Others in their environment should be encouraged to use the My Pain Alert ^{TM} Scale to demonstrate its use, expressing their request for pain relief.

Relate elements of the boy's story to the individual's environment. Do they have over-the - counter medications? What do those meds look like? Where is the water they use to take them? Do they watch cartoons with a character who gets hurt? What level of pain should the character point to? Do they have a "going to the hospital" story book? What does the character experience? What pain level might the character point to?

Using the limited communicator's daily routine can help with the time concepts involved. If they take other medicines, when do they take them? When do they need more? Do they understand the time it takes for the medicine to take effect? Talk about the route the medicine takes in their body. Talk about when their body needs more of the medicine. What activities are associated with times for medications?

Practice before need is important to get these ideas across to the very young or limited communicator. When they are hurting, they may **not be able** to focus on anything new.

The first use of My Pain Alert ™ Scale with the individual in pain may go like this:

The caregiver makes a guess as to the severity level of pain. Resource websites in the Brief Annotated Bibliography may help with this guess. The caregiver reads the boy's story about one level higher, then reads the story material about the "best guess" level. Then pointing at the scale pictures, the caregiver asks: Does your pain feel like this boy or that boy?

Giving the choice twice and getting two responses increases the reliability of the individual's response. If the response is unclear, then the caregiver should choose the **lower** level saying: "I think you feel like this boy. I'm going to help you show me, then give you (medication)." The caregiver takes the individual's hand and points to the appropriate level picture.

Praise the individual for their efforts to use the scale.

Continue with the page about taking medicine. After a short time, observation may show that the **dose is inadequate**, yet time is needed before an alternative is tried. The caregiver can model and encourage actions: take deep relaxing breaths, provide a light massage, reduce noise and distraction in the environment, or snuggle in bed with a soft blanket. As these actions are taken **tell the individual that you know they are hurting,** and relate their experience to the appropriate level story. This validates the individual's effort to communicate, justifying another effort at another time.

My Pain Alert ™ Stories

Describe each pain level

Level 1   Ouch!

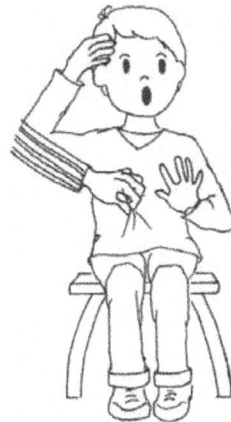

See the boy being pinched in his belly. He says: "Ouch!"
The hurt does not last. His mother might kiss it to make him feel better.
She could give him a hug and say: "You are okay now."

Have you been pinched?   Did it hurt? What picture would you point to? What if you bumped
your head?   What if you stubbed your toe? What picture would tell how you feel? The pain is
Level one – Ouch!

Communication
Tool

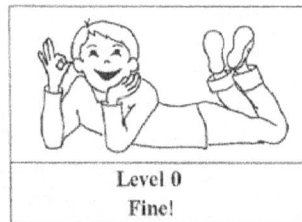

Level 0
Fine!

My Pain Alert ™ Scale

By
Gail Goldstein, CCC-SLP, Speech Therapist
Jan Schippits, Marketing, Illustration, Design,
Blair Malloy, Music, Use, Photo Consultant
Copyright 2016

| Level 1 Ouch! | Level 2 Need Meds! | Level 3 Need Stronger! | Level 4 Meds Not Working! | Level 5 Need Escape! |

Level 2   Need Meds!

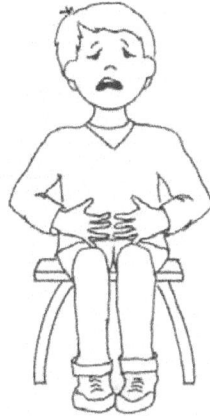

See this boy. He groans: "Oh...oh...oh." He is holding his belly because it hurts. The hurt does not go away. He needs help to feel better. His mother can give him children's acetaminophen. She will look at him carefully, weigh him and read the directions before measuring it out.

Have you ever felt like that? What picture would you point to?
Have you had a headache and wanted it to go away? What picture would you point to?
Over-the-counter medicine taken with a glass of water can help the pain go away.

This medicine will wear out with time. If the boy hurts the same way, he will need more. What picture should he point to? When his mother checks on him she may say, "You took medicine before breakfast. Now it's after lunch, and the medicine doesn't always last this long. How are you? Do you need more meds to make you feel fine again?" What picture should the boy point to letting her know he needs more of the same medicine? The pain is Level Two – Need Meds!

Communication Tool

Level 0
Fine!

My Pain Alert ™ Scale

By
Gail Goldstein, CCC-SLP, Speech Therapist
Jan Schippits, Marketing, Illustration, Design,
Blair Malloy, Music, Use, Photo Consultant
Copyright 2016

Level 1	Level 2	Level 3	Level 4	Level 5
Ouch!	Need Meds!	Need Stronger!	Meds Not Working!	Need Escape!

Take Medicine!

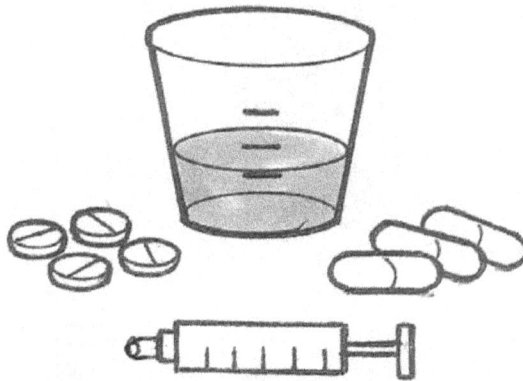

Do you have over-the-counter medicine? Is it a liquid to drink, a pill, or a capsule? Point to the kind of medicine you can take. What color is it? What is it called? The tablets or shiny capsules need to float down your throat, like they are surfing a water wave. The amount of medicine you take depends on your size. Each day you change a little, so each time you need medicine, it is good to check the directions before you take it, so you get exactly the right amount for your size.

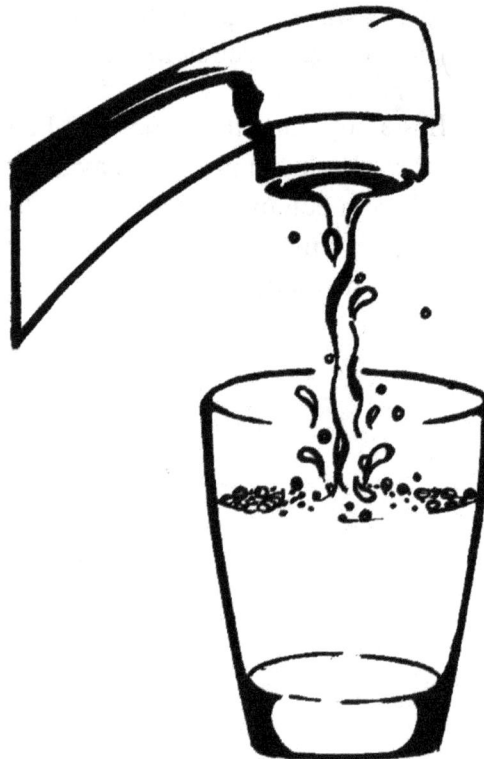

Here is the water to drink coming from a faucet. Some water comes from bottles. Water speeds the medicine on its way to fight the pain. You can drink a lot of water to make the medicine work as fast as it can. Some medicine works best when taken with food like applesauce or bread. The food helps the medicine work well. Knowing how to take medicine is important. Does the medicine you can take go with water or with food and water?

Level 0   Fine!

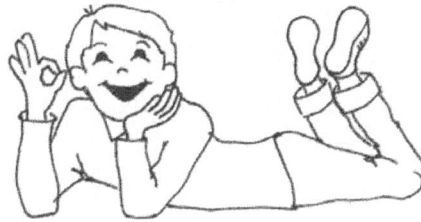

See the boy lying on his belly. After his mother gave him medicine, and it started to work, he felt fine. He is okay now and can rest on the part of his belly that hurt before taking meds. He is telling his mother that the medicine worked by making the okay sign with his hand.   He can also smile and say, "I am fine now." Which boy below is fine? Point to the boy who feels good and is fine. The no pain level is Level 0 – Fine!

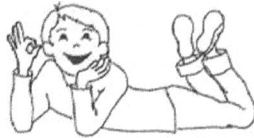

Communication Tool

Level 0
Fine!

My Pain Alert ™ Scale

By
Gail Goldstein, CCC-SLP, Speech Therapist
Jan Schippits, Marketing, Illustration, Design,
Blair Malloy, Music, Use, Photo Consultant
Copyright 2016

Level 1	Level 2	Level 3	Level 4	Level 5
Ouch!	Need Meds!	Need Stronger!	Meds Not Working!	Need Escape!

Level 3   Need Stronger Meds!

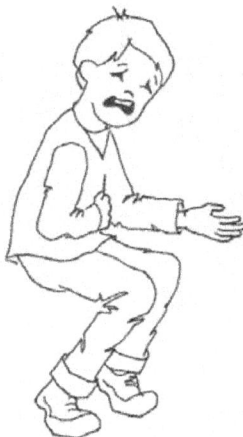

See the boy holding his sore belly and reaching out for help. He hurts. He moans: "Ehh...ehh...eh." The over-the-counter medicine was not strong enough. He took the medicine and waited. It did not take all the pain away. He still hurts. He is asking for stronger medicine.

Only some people need stronger medicine for pain. The boy's doctor would know what could help him. Do you know someone who gets special medicine from the doctor to help them hurt less? What picture would they point to if they needed stronger medicine for pain? Does this boy need regular pain medicine or stronger medicine for pain? Point to the boy who needs stronger medicine. The pain is Level 3 – Need Stronger Meds!

Communication Tool

Level 0
Fine!

My Pain Alert ™ **Scale**

By
Gail Goldstein, CCC-SLP, Speech Therapist
Jan Schippits, Marketing, Illustration, Design,
Blair Malloy, Music, Use, Photo Consultant
Copyright 2016

| Level 1 Ouch! | Level 2 Need Meds! | Level 3 Need Stronger! | Level 4 Meds Not Working! | Level 5 Need Escape! |

Level 4   Meds Not Working!

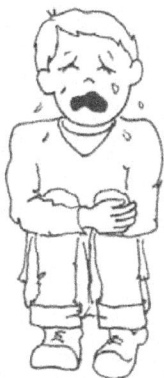

See the boy crying: "Uh…sniff…uh…sniff…uh." He hurts a lot! The stronger medicine for his pain is not working. He needs more help for his pain. His mother asks him to look at the pictures on the next page and tell about his pain: is it sharp, dull, throbbing or burning? Where did it start? Is it in another place on his body now? Is it growing more painful? He tells her and she writes it down, then calls the doctor. She asks for help because the boy's pain is very bad. Point to the boy who is crying because his pain is very bad. The pain is Level 4 – Meds Not Working!

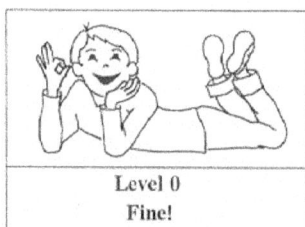

Communication Tool

Level 0
Fine!

My Pain Alert ™ Scale

By
Gail Goldstein, CCC-SLP, Speech Therapist
Jan Schippits, Marketing, Illustration, Design,
Blair Malloy, Music, Use, Photo Consultant
Copyright 2016

Level 1 Ouch!	Level 2 Need Meds!	Level 3 Need Stronger!	Level 4 Meds Not Working!	Level 5 Need Escape!

Where Does It Hurt?

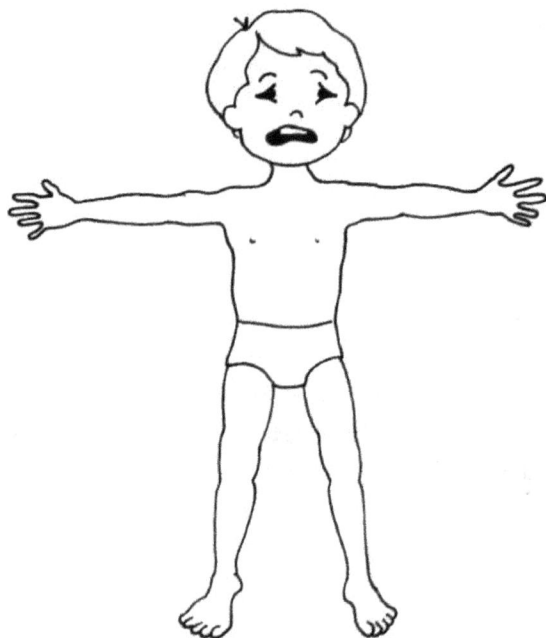

Point to the place on the boy where you hurt.

Touch the spots where your body hurts.

How Does It Hurt?

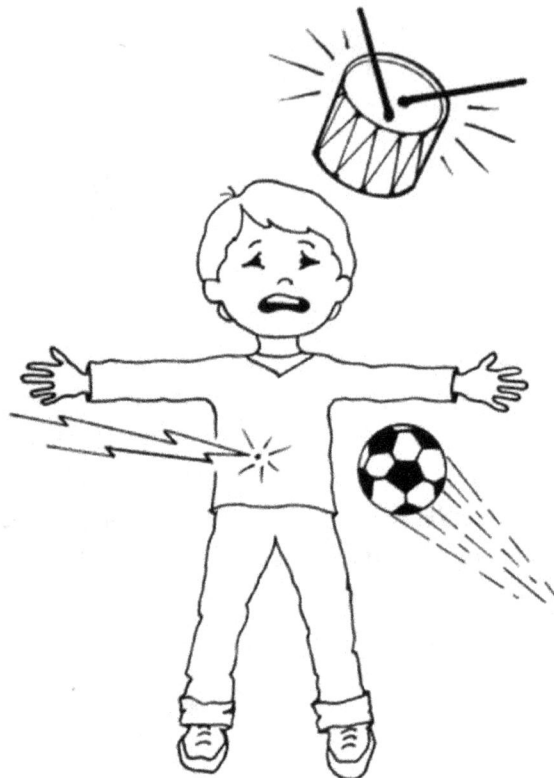

Does it hurt like a beating drum?
Boom Boom Boom!
Does it hurt like a sharp point?
Does it hurt like a big ball pushing on you?

How Much Does it Hurt?

If the dark circle is before, how big is your pain now?

Does the pain feel like it is **grow*ing*?**

Level 5   Need Escape!

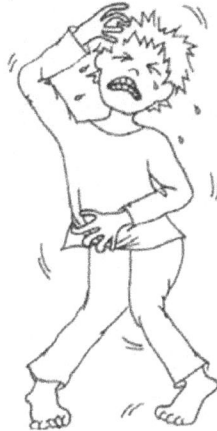

See the boy biting down hard with his teeth and crying. See him twisting his body. He is making a noise: "EEEEEEEE" on each breath. He hurts so bad that he tosses and turns his body to try to get some relief from the pain. The medicines that were tried for his pain are not working. The boy's pain is very, very bad. He would not mind a needle injection or medicine through a tube into his body, if it helped the pain go away. He would like to be unconscious so that he can escape the pain. He needs more help from the doctor, because his pain hurts more than he can tolerate. He says, "Do something so I don't feel the pain." Point to the boy who needs help because he has pain that hurts more than he can stand. This pain is Level 5 - Need Escape!

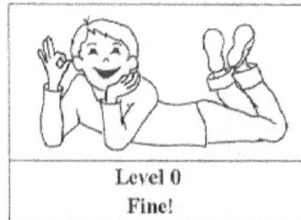

Communication
Tool

Level 0
Fine!

My Pain Alert ™ Scale

By
Gail Goldstein, CCC-SLP, Speech Therapist
Jan Schippits, Marketing, Illustration, Design,
Blair Malloy, Music, Use, Photo Consultant
Copyright 2016

Level 1	Level 2	Level 3	Level 4	Level 5
Ouch!	Need Meds!	Need Stronger!	Meds Not Working!	Need Escape!

American Sign Language

Use this question and cues from the pain level stories to elicit ASL responses for each of the My Pain Alert ™ Scale levels.

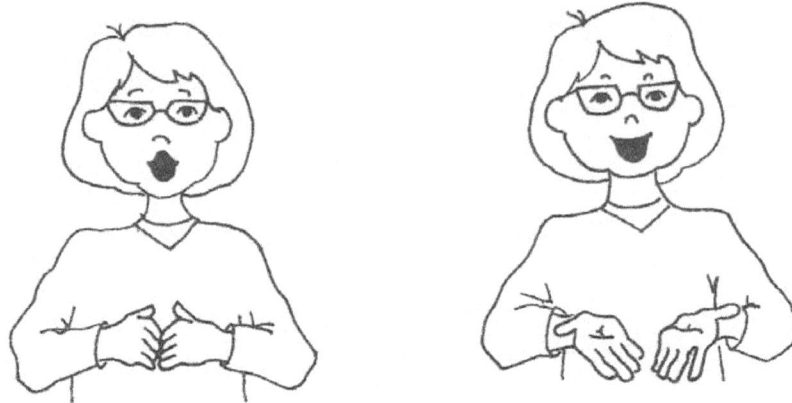

How Are - Start with Right angle hands palms down and knuckles touching, then swing them up and open to the palms up position.

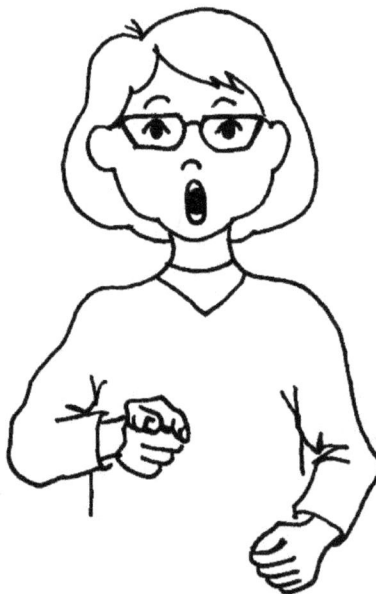

You ? – Then Right index finger points to person being asked.

Ouch! Level 1   ASL Signs

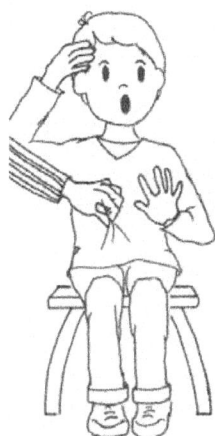

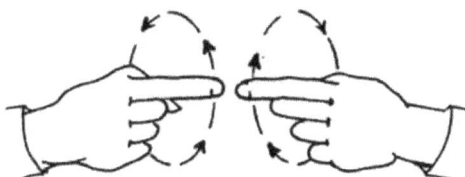

Pain - "d" hand pointing fingers circle elliptically in opposite directions in front of chest.

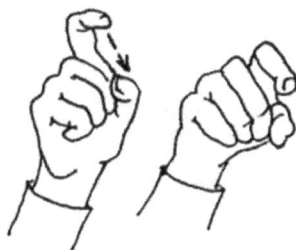

Need - Right "x" hand moves forcefully up and down once or twice.

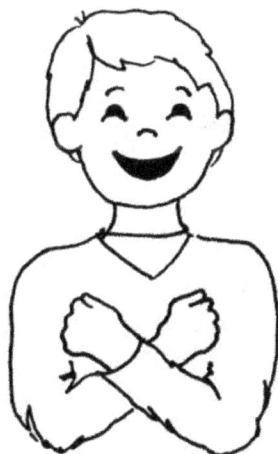

Hug - Crossed arms clasp body in hugging position.

Need Meds! Level 2   ASL Sign

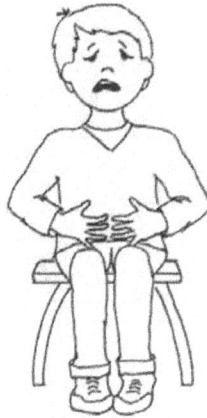

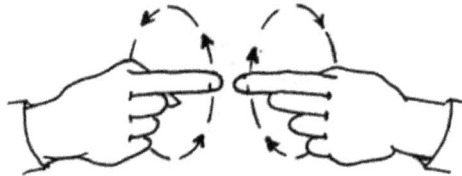

Pain - "d" hand pointing fingers circle elliptically in opposite directions in front of chest.

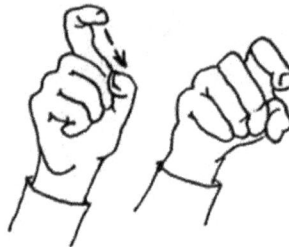

Need - Right "x" hand moves forcefully up and down once or twice.

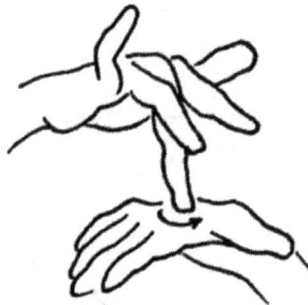

Medicine - Right middle fingertip makes small counterclockwise circles in upturned Left palm.

Take Medicine!

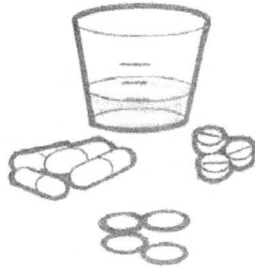

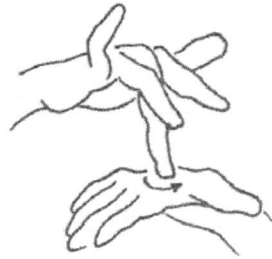

Medicine - Right middle fingertip makes small counterclockwise circles in Left palm.

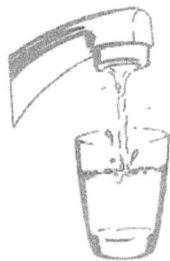

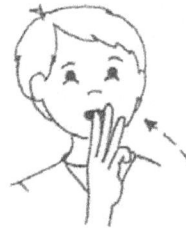

Water – Touch Right index finger of "w" hand to mouth once or twice.

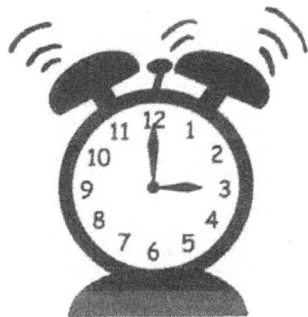

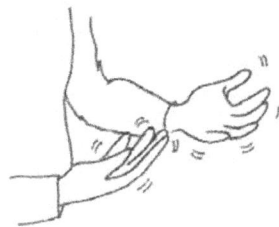

Wait – Hold both curved open palm up hands to Left. Wiggle fingers.

Fine! Level 0 ASL Sign

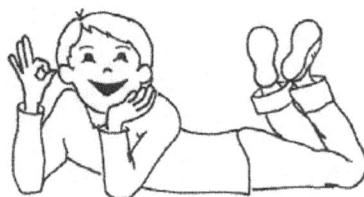

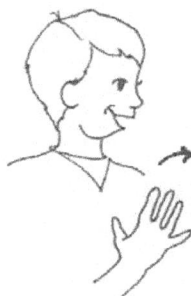

Fine - Put thumb of open Right hand to chest, then move hand up and forward.

Need Strong Meds! Level 3   ASL Sign

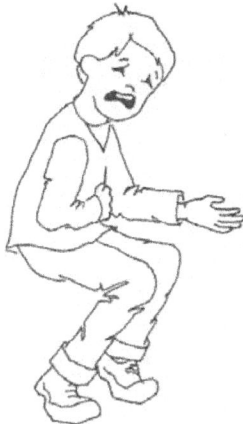

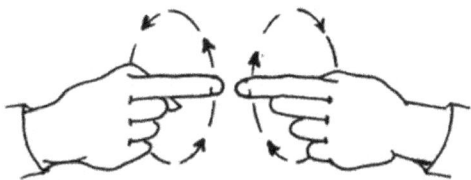

Pain – "d" hand pointing fingers circle elliptically in opposite directions in front of chest.

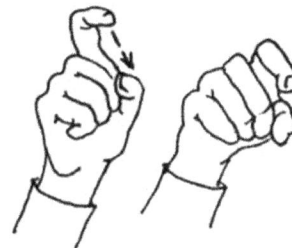

Need – Right "x" hand moves forcefully up and down once or twice.

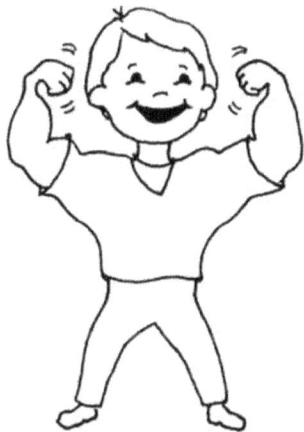

Strong - Make muscles shaking fists.

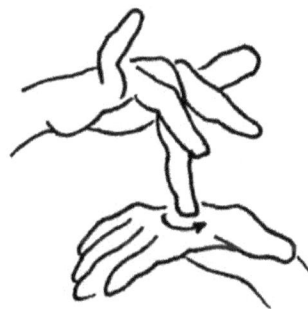

Medicine – Right middle fingertip makes small counterclockwise circles in Left palm.

Meds Not Working! Level 4   ASL Sign

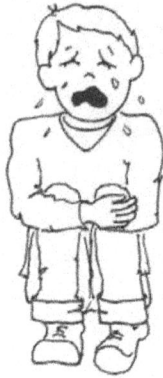

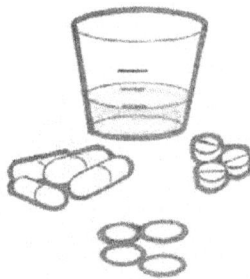

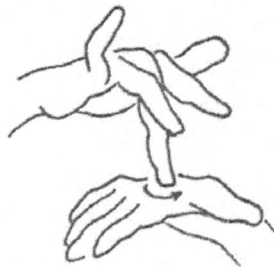

Medicine – Right middle fingertip makes small counterclockwise circles in Left palm.

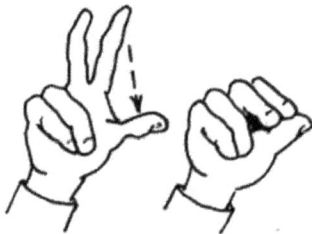

No – Bring Right thumb, index, and middle finger together.

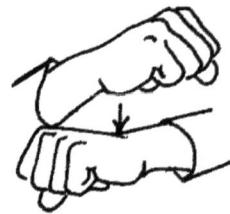

Work – Tap wrist of Right fist on wrist of Left fist a few times.

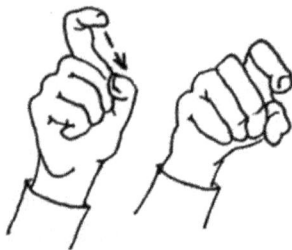

Need- Right "x" hand moves forcefully up and down once or twice.

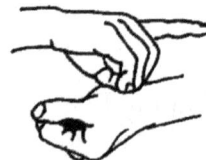

Doctor - Place Right "d" hand fingers down on on Left wrist.

Need Escape! Level 5   ASL Sign

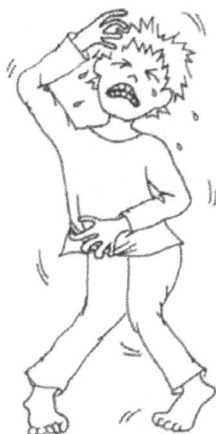

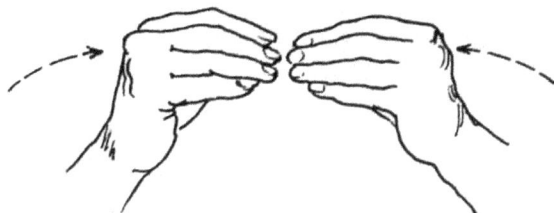

More – Right hand comes up to meet Left in front of chest. Touch fingertips of both hands with palms down, thumbs touching fingers of same hand.

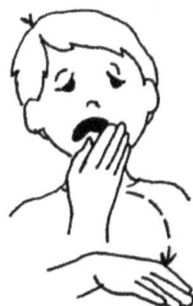

Bad – Fingertips of Right flat hand at lips, then move it so palm faces down by waist.

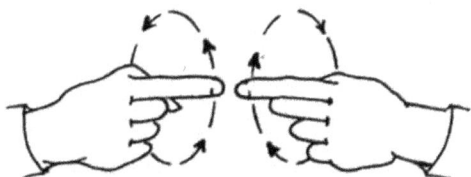

Pain – "d" hands pointing fingers circle elliptically in opposite directions in front of chest.

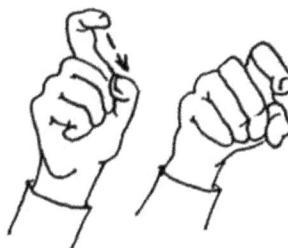

Need – Right "x" hand moves force-fully up and down once or twice.

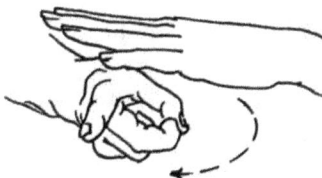

Escape – Downturned Left hand covers downturned Right "d" hand. Then Right "d" hand moves quickly right and away.

Are You Hurting? My Pain Alert ™ Song

Individual starts verse by voicing sounds paired with that verse and acting it out. These sounds are included to make this tool useful to those with verbal apraxia, an inability to reproduce the complex oral muscle movement patterns of words.

1. Ouch!
2. Oh! Oh! Oh
3. Eh! Eh! Ehh!
4. Uh! Sniff Uh!
5. EEEEE EEE!

Caregiver sings the question and individual points to the appropriate picture on the
My Pain Alert ™ Scale.

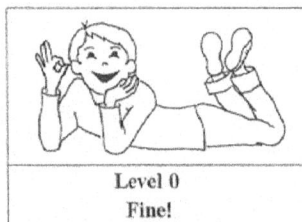

Communication Tool	Level 0 Fine!

My Pain Alert ™ Scale

By
Gail Goldstein, CCC-SLP, Speech Therapist
Jan Schippits, Marketing, Illustration, Design,
Blair Malloy, Music, Use, Photo Consultant
Copyright 2016

Level 1 Ouch!	Level 2 Need Meds!	Level 3 Need Stronger!	Level 4 Meds Not Working!	Level 5 Need Escape!

Individual may act out the remainder of each verse as it is sung using a different type of pain for each practice: headache, foot pain, shoulder pain, etc.

Are You Hurting? My Pain Alert™ Song

Lyrics: Gail Goldstein Music: Blair Malloy

1. Ouch! Are you hurt ing my dear one? Let me see, let me feel, just a shock that

felt so real. Here's a hug, and so you're done. Now you go back to having fun!

REFRAIN: I'm check ing on you. Now it's time. Are you hurting? Are you fine?

2. Oh! Oh! Need Meds! (groan)   Are you hurt ing my dear one?   Let me see, let me feel,
3. Eh! Eh! Need Stronger (moan)   Are you hurt ing my dear one?   Let me see, let me feel,
4. Uh! Sniff Uh! Meds Not Working (cry) Are you hurt ing my dear one?   Let me see, let me feel,
5. EE! EEE! Need Escape! (hysterical)   Are you hurt ing my dear one?   Let me see, let me feel,

2. Need to know how we can deal   A chy hot or very   sore,   We'll read and check before I pour.
3. Need to know how we can deal   Here's your meds. We'll pour out some. Now drink some water while I hum.
4. Need to know what helps to heal. Where's the pain? Please show me all. We'll write it down and make a call.
5. Need to know what helps to heal.   So much pain.   Please show me where. You need to have some special care.

2. Water helps the meds to go   To the pain that hurts you so. Breathe deep and rest, You know I'm here.
3. Water helps the meds to go   To the pain that hurts you so. Breathe deep and rest, You know I'm here.
4. We'll call the doctors, they will know: What to do and where to go. Breathe deep and rest, You know I'm here.
5. We'll call the doctors, they will know: What to do and where to go. Breathe deep and rest, You know I'm here.

Brief Annotated Bibliography

Brief Annotated Bibliography for My Pain Alert ™ Scale Communication Tool

Bahan, Ben and Joe Dannis. *Signs for Me Basic Sign Vocabulary for Children, Parents & Teachers.* San Diego, CA: Dawn Sign Press, 1990. Print.

City of Hope Pain & Palliative Care Resource Center. *Categories of Materials. IV. Pain and Symptom Management. A. Pain Assessment Tools.* Modified February 1, 2016. www.prc.coh/pain_assessment.asp Web. Accessed March 30, 2016.

Drager, Kathryn D. R. "Aided Modeling Interventions for Children with Autism Spectrum Disorders Who Require AAC." *SIG 12 Perspectives on Augmentative and Alternative Communication.* Volume 18 (December 2009): 114-120. www.asha.org Web. Accessed March 27, 2016. "This article discusses the research evidence suggesting that aided modeling interventions may be effective for children with autism spectrum disorders (ASD)."

FDA, Department of Health and Human Services, U.S. Food and Drug Administration. *Medicines In My Home information for students on the safe use of over-the-counter medicines.* Publication No. (FDA) 07-1906. www.fda.gov/medsinmyhome Web. Accessed March 27, 2016.

Flodin, Mickey. *Signing for Kids.* New York, NY: Perigee Books, 1991. Print.

Hasselkus, Amy. "Health Communication: Implications for Diverse Populations." *SIG 14 Perspectives on Communication Disorders and Sciences in Culturally and Linguistically Diverse Populations.* Volume 18 (March 2011): 12-19. www.asha.org Web. Accessed March 27, 2016. "…poor health literacy has been estimated to cost between $106-238 billion each year. Health literacy also contributes to health disparities."

Komesidou, Rouzana and Holly L. Storkel. "Learning and Remembering New Words: Clinical Illustrations from Children with Specific Language Impairment." *SIG 1 Perspectives on Language Learning and Education.* Volume 22 (November 2015): 138-146. www.asha.org Web. Accessed March 27, 2016. "…at least two neurocognitive processes involved in word learning: a) learning from input and b) memory evolution in the absence of input."

Rao, Paul R. "Our Role in Effective Parent-Provider Communication." *The Asha Leader.* Volume 16 (November 2011): 17. www.asha.org Web. Accessed March 27, 2016. "Based on data from NIH and MarkeTrak VII estimates of "communication-vulnerable individuals…in health care settings in the United States…is more than two-thirds of the entire population." "Anyone entering the health care system should have services and tools available to allow them to communicate with health care professionals."

Roberts, Megan Y. and Ann P. Kaiser. "The Effectiveness of Parent-Implemented Language Interventions: A Meta-Analysis." *American Journal of Speech-Language Pathology.* Volume 20 (August 2011): 180-199. www.asha.org Web. Accessed March 27, 2016. "The results of this review indicate that parent-implemented language interventions are an effective approach to early language intervention for young children with language impairments."

Brief Annotated Bibliography for My Pain Alert ™ Scale Communication Tool continued

Spencer, Trina D., Douglas B. Petersen and John L. Adams. "Tier 2 Language Intervention for Diverse Preschoolers: An Early Stage Randomized Control Group Study Following an Analysis of Response to Intervention." *American Journal of Speech Language Pathology*. Volume 24 (November 2015): 619-635. www.asha.org Web. Accessed March 27, 2016. "…evidence that narrative language intervention is an effective approach to improving language skills of preschoolers with diverse language needs."

Steinberg, Martin L. *American Sign Language Concise Dictionary.* New York, NY: Harper and Row Publishers, 1990. Print.

"Tell me how it hurts." *Consumer Reports Magazine* (June 2016): 30-31. Print.

Verghise, Susan T. and Raafat S. Hannallah. "Acute Pain Management in Children." *Journal of Pain Management* (July 2010): 105-123. "…factors such as fear, anxiety, coping style, and lack of social support can further aggravate physical pain in children." www.ncbi.nlm.nih.gov >PMC3004641 Accessed May 13, 2016.

Voelme, Krista and Holly L. Storkel. "Teaching New Words to Children with Specific Language Impairment." *SIG 1 Perspectives on Language Learning and Education.* Volume 22 (November 2015): 131-137. www.asha.org Web. Accessed March 27, 2016. "…review of evidence base for interactive book reading to facilitate new word learning for preschool and school age children," "children with Specific Language Impairment need 2-3 times as many exposures as typically developing children to learn new words." "Current results suggest that 36 story retelling exposures is the most promising intensity for children with SLI."

Walsh, Trudi M., Patrick J. McGrath and Douglas K. Symons. "Attachment dimensions and young children's response to pain." *Pain Research and Management* Volume 13 #1 (January/February 2008): 33-40. www.ncbi.nim.nih.gov Web . Accessed March 13, 2016.

Wilner, L. Scott and Robert Arnold. *Fast Facts and Concepts: #126 Pain Assessment in the Cognitively Impaired.* Palliative Care Network of Wisconsin. www.mypcnw.org Web. Accessed March 27, 2016.

Wong, Donna L. and Connie M. Baker. "Pain in Children: Comparison of Assessment Scales." *Pediatric Nursing* Volume 14 #1 (January-February 1988) www.wongbakerfaces.org Web. Accessed March 29, 2016.

Yorkston, Kathryn M., Carolyn R. Baylor and Michael I. Burns. "Stimulating Patient Communication Strategies." *The ASHA Leader* Volume 21 (March 2016): 46-51. www.asha.org Web. Accessed March 27, 2016. "Medical students practice 'FRAME' strategies" paraphrased: F = familiarize with communication strategies patient prefers or requires, R= reduce speaking rate, A= assist with communication, M= mix communication methods, and E= engage the patient.

TOOLS

Recommended Data Standardization

Caregiver Notes To Support Medical Care

Note Page

My Pain Alert ™ Scale

Recommended Data Standardization

The creators of this tool are loved ones with strong skill sets and no current professional affiliation with care provision agencies. Many studies in many settings are needed to give a tool like this "gold standard" traction. So, with all due respect to the professionals in hospitals, clinics, rehabilitation agencies, schools, and sheltered care settings, below are some questions to facilitate "in house" quality assurance in regard to patient pain communication. Our hope is to have some consistency across data sets from different studies. This consistency will enable decisive meta-studies to be published clarifying this tool's validity and reliability, as well as your cost impact of improving patient pain communication.

A second goal is to facilitate single subject studies as there are many people with unique combinations of disorders needing scientific attention and many advanced students in need of single subject studies to perfect their clinical and research skills. We encourage therapeutic professionals in training to use the following in their data sets as well.

Question for admitting, start of new year, or change of personnel dealing primarily with this limited communicator, mark as many as apply:
1. How does patient express pain at home? _____ meets own needs without other's help; _____ tells caregiver with words like "hurt", "pain", "ouch"; ____uses a pain scale; _____ uses assisted communication device: ____ face shows distress; ____ squirms, body actions; ___ cries; ____ points. Use lines below to detail communication device history, and/or pain scale practice log, and/or other method: _____

_____

Questions for release from facility, end of year, or end of primary personnel's responsibility (filled out by personnel named and signed below):
1. Limited communicator's communication of pain is: _____clear and consistent, _____ adequate, _____inconsistent or questionable:_____
2. If questionable or inconsistent, were facility operations effected: ____patient required more staff time to get needs met; _____patient's reaction to pain resulted in injury (_patient or_ staff); ____patient's reaction to pain resulted in material waste; _____patient care was less than ideal.
3. If patient response was adequate, inconsistent or questionable: What helped? _____

_____
What hindered? _____
4. Was a pain scale used? _____ Name of scale_____
5. Practice with scale prior to use with pain: _____none, ____1-5 sessions, ____6-10 sessions, _____ 11-20 sessions, _____21-36 sessions, _____37 or more sessions, _____unknown.
6. Family/caregivers were present during ____ percent of personnel's interaction with patient.
7. _____percent of observed interactions family/caregivers appeared supportive of patient.
8. ____percent of observed interactions family/caregivers appeared supportive of treatment plan.
Comments:_____

_____

Signature_____Name_____Date_____

Notes to Support Medical Care

The effectiveness of My Pain Alert™ Scale is dependent on the limited communicator having practice with the stories for each level to learn the differences between the levels. The e-book format allows the caregiver to use the "Notes" function on their viewing device (smart phone, tablet, computer) to record notes about what was practiced, and how the individual responded. A record of what happened each practice time can then be shared with medical and communication professionals. Details "at the time of pain" about the individual's behaviors and responses are valuable. The record can provide important clues as to what is needed to improve the life quality of the limited communicator.

To make this important record keeping task easy, here is a quick way to write these notes. These are the elements that are needed:

   At the top: User Identification(name):
                User age in years ____-months_____ on **date of first look** at the stories.

   Date of practice or use: Year, Month, Day

   Use a letter **P** for a practice session and a **U** or "Use" for actual use with a pain experience.

   Tell what was included in the practice or use experience:
      Boy's Stories: **bs**
      American Sign Language responses: **asl**
      Are you Hurting? song melody: **m**
      My Pain Alert ™ Scale: **scale**

   List the levels which were attended to by the individual during practice. If you read all the stories but your individual closed their eyes or got distracted during the last two you would record: 1,2,0,3. If you finished all the stories record: **120345**. If you finished stories, and some ASL signs record: 120345 (or **all**) + **ASL 1203**

   How did individual respond: pointing, speaking, ASL signing, other gestures, making sounds, attending? **Write this part out**.

   Your assessment of the person's response: Was it great, good, okay, distracted, possible seizure, or other intervening condition? This is another place where your detail is important.

   If the experience was a **Use** of the scale, what was the result?

Examples:

Here are some examples of Notes using this format:
Date -- Which materials used – Levels covered-- Patient's response methods-- Response quality, Result:
Joey 2years 7 months
2016,March 4th, **P,bs,m,scale**, 120345, point, speak, good, appeared to be learning.
2016,March 8th, **P,bs,asl,scale**, 1203, point, sounds, tried some signs, good, signs are hard to do.
2016,March 15th, **U, m, scale**, 203 repeated three times, point, sounds, facial expression, fussy actions, might be 'flu. Attended to song melody and responded. Dose of acetaminophen appeared right for relieving discomfort.
Set up notes page like this:

_____

My Pain Alert TM Scale and Stories

Notes for _____ Age _____ on Start Date _____

Date * P or U * Elements * Levels * Individual's Responses * Caregiver's Impressions

My Pain Alert ™ Scale

By
Gail Goldstein, CCC-SLP, Speech Therapist
Jan Schippits, Marketing, Illustration, Design,
Blair Malloy, Music, Use, Photo Consultant
Copyright 2016

Communication Tool

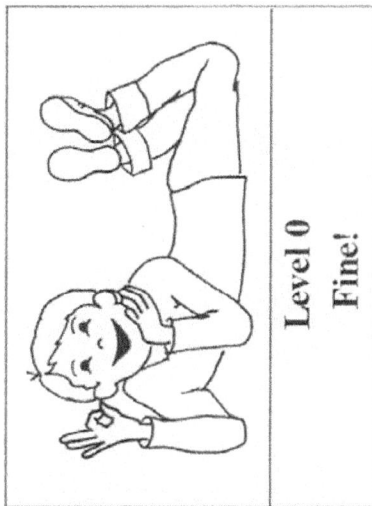

Level 0 Fine!

Level 1 Ouch!	Level 2 Need Meds!	Level 3 Need Stronger!	Level 4 Meds Not Working!	Level 5 Need Escape!

www.ingramcontent.com/pod-product-compliance
Lightning Source LLC
Chambersburg PA
CBHW080401030426
42334CB00024B/2959